APPLE CIDER VINEGAR

THE MIRACLE APPLE CIDER VINEGAR SOLUTION FOR WEIGHT LOSS, DIGESTIVE HEALTH & BEAUTIFUL SKIN

Jessica Jacobs

information is without contract or any type of guarantee assurance.

The trademarks that are used are without any consent, and the publication of the trademark is without permission or backing by the trademark owner. All trademarks and brands within this book are for clarifying purposes only and are the owned by the owners themselves, not affiliated with this document.

INTRODUCTION

This book contains proven steps and strategies on how to use apple cider vinegar in your everyday life to lose weight, maintain beautiful skin and good health, and attain many other goals.

Have you noticed how many alternative treatments are out there? The current generation seems to be evermore appreciative of the vast benefits of using unconventional treatments such as juice fasts and extreme diets– like the paleo diet– to lose weight and achieve other goals. All these are great alternative treatments that can help you achieve the respective goals. The problem is that all of them require strong willpower, sacrifice, time and money to execute effectively if you are to be one of the success stories that you desperately want to be. With so many of these recommendations and tips available, it can make one feel overwhelmed in choosing the proper regimen to follow. Do you know that you don't have to do all that in order to lose weight, detoxify your body and achieve many other goals that are important to you? Then it's time to test out a very common substance that you can even find in your kitchen. It's all in the humble apple cider. Forget about expensive and possibly harmful concoctions that might just waste your effort and money. This book will unearth the effectiveness of apple cider vinegar in promoting weight loss and better hair, skin and general health.

Thanks again for downloading this book, I hope you enjoy it!

Table of Contents

APPLE CIDER VINEGAR: AN INTRODUCTION

Ever tried that sour and tangy with a distinct acidic smell and taste that is just quite difficult for some to get used to? That's apple cider. A delicious drink for some which is made from crushed apples. In another form, you've probably heard about apple cider vinegar and its many benefits, but do you know where it comes from, what it does, how it works, and how to use it? This book will answer those questions and introduce you to the possible uses of apple cider vinegar to achieve benefits including weight loss, skin and hair care, health maintenance, a more sanitary home, and many others you probably didn't know about.

Apple Cider Vinegar: What is it?

Vinegar has been around since the olden times and was used throughout history for a variety of purposes including killing weeds, polishing armor, cleaning coffee makers, making pickles, dressing salads, cosmetic needs and treating various diseases. All over the world and across many cultures, there are many so many types of vinegar made from different types of food that underwent a process called "fermentation". It is mainly comprised by a mixture of acetic acid and water. It is a prized culinary ingredient with a mild, sour and acidic taste that adds exquisite flavor to certain dishes. Among the many types of vinegar, the most exceptional according to natural practitioners is the vinegar derived from apples. Apple cider vinegar (ACV for short), made from cider or apple must, is believed to be the most effective type of vinegar for treating a wide variety of medical conditions. This has given it a worldwide following, and its culinary uses include marinades, salad dressings, food preservatives, vinaigrettes and chutneys, to name just a few. Its color ranges from medium yellowish brown to pale amber. Organic, unfiltered, unpasteurized ACV (which is the healthiest kind) is translucent or foggy in appearance because it contains "mother of vinegar". This is a combination of acetic acid bacteria and a type of cellulose, and is a byproduct of the fermentation of alcohol into acetic acid in the presence of oxygen. Although mother of vinegar may not look appetizing, it is harmless.

With so many potential uses of apple cider vinegar for your kitchen recipes, in the household and in the realm of medicinal practice, then it is not unlikely that you need not look far for other possible applications of the apple cider vinegar.

CHAPTER 1:
HOW CAN APPLE CIDER VINEGAR BE OF USE TO YOU?

Apple cider vinegar was used as folk remedy long before it started growing popular in the US during the 1950s.People around the world, who tried the substance have reported health benefits including reversal of the aging process, improvement in digestion, and detoxification, as well as other uses such as being an effective flea control on pets. While not all of the claims have been scientifically verified, a number of them have, and it's hard to overlook the growing popularity of the 'miracle cure liquid'. Different people experience different levels of success with ACV, so trying it yourself is the best way find out what benefits you'll obtain.

The next section explores the secrets of using ACV for weight loss, more beautiful skin and a myriad of other applications in the home. Remember, an apple a day keeps the doctor away— and that may be even more true if the apple is in the form of vinegar!

Why so? The process of fermentation that gives the apple cider vinegar its sour taste and distinct smell is made possible by bacteria and yeast that first convert sugar into alcohol then to acetic acid which gives the characteristics of ACV as we know it. Worried about the bacteria, you say? Fear not because the organisms acting in the process of ACV fermentation is nonetheless healthy and very beneficial to the human body. As an end product, the liquid produced from fermented apples is full of minerals like magnesium, sodium, chloride, phosphorus, potassium, calcium, and even trace minerals including fluorine, copper, plus vitamins A, B1, B2, B6, C, and

E, bioflavonoid, and pectin. Indeed ACV is a healthy elixir for the body and no other type of vinegar is as healthy and comparable to it.

CHAPTER 2:
USE APPLE CIDER VINEGAR FOR WEIGHT LOSS AND DETOXIFICATION

WEIGHT LOSS

You may be one of the many people all over the world who have spent conscious efforts into trying effective means of reducing your total body mass. So you have you subjected yourself to any of the following; killer diets; really expensive equipment; fat burning pills; and so many other techniques that never truly worked? And all of it brought negative feelings of expectation despite your efforts? Then here is good news! You might just have found the easiest alternative available to man. If you have been struggling to lose weight for years, apple cider vinegar could be part of the solution to successfully regain that ideal body you've been dying to have. Well technically speaking, it is best not to have extremely high expectations if you cannot fully follow a strict weight loss method. Yet there is assurance that incorporating this weight reduction elixir in your lifestyle habits can indeed help you shed some pounds in a gradual manner. There are countless success stories of people who have shed up to fifteen pounds a year while drinking just one or two tablespoons of ACV daily. This is the amount of weight you can reduce at a more reasonable pace. This is also that rate of weight loss which is a lot more realistic than losing fifteen pounds in just two weeks while on a juice fast or low-carb diet. And it's a lot easier to take a couple of spoonfuls of ACV than it is to spend a couple of hours at the gym or fast for weeks. Even better, the weight-loss effect has been proven scientifically. A 2005 study showed that people who consumed small amounts of vinegar with their meals felt fuller than those who didn't when eating the same quantity of food. In another study conducted in 2009, people who consumed acetic acid daily over a 12-week period experienced a significant decrease in waist circumference, abdominal fat, triglycerides, and body weight. So what's in the ACV that causes weight loss, and how does it work? Read on for the answer . . .

The acidic nature of ACV and iron production

You can never guess how beneficial ACV is to the proper utilization of iron in the human body. With iron, properly processed, the immune system which protects the body from diseases and infections is strengthened to a healthy state and enable the repair by connective tissues in the body. In this case, the acidity in apple cider vinegar releases iron from the foods you eat, making it available when needed. As a necessary protein, iron is processed in the blood. It can be taken from the foods you consume or even in the form of nutritional iron supplement. Iron is an important component of myoglobin and hemoglobin, which supply oxygen to your cells. Your cells use the oxygen to burn calories. Thus, when the body gets more iron, the oxygen supply increases, and burning calories is a lot easier. That obviously helps greatly with weight loss. A tablespoon or two of ACV daily is enough to help proper iron metabolism contributing to a non-drastic but healthy pace of weight reduction. It is just safe and effective posing little to no risk if used properly as a supplement.

Presence of pectin in apple cider vinegar

Apple cider vinegar contains pectin, a naturally occurring thickening agent that expands when mixed with water in the stomach. It is this benefit of apple cider vinegar that can help suppress appetite. When pectin thickens a reaction in the stomach will trigger an expansion which will provide signals to the brain that you no longer need food as much food to consume. This expansion which occurs in the digestive tract makes you feel fuller, leaving you satisfied for longer and less susceptible to overeating or snacking because of hunger pangs or cravings. Pectin, found in apples from which ACV is made, is really beneficial to the body not only because it is a good antioxidant which lowers bad cholesterol, but also regulates the digestive system due to the high amount of fiber. It is also water soluble and can absorb harmful wastes such as fat, bad cholesterol, to name a few and contributing to the effective flushing of these harmful radicals out of the body system. Overall the presence of pectin improves the overall performance of your heart as well as your digestive tract.

Apple cider vinegar contains potassium

Do you love bananas as much as I do? It is a scientific fact that it has the sweet, yellow, firm and curved body that makes it the world's most popular fruit. And such popularity of banana all over the globe is not attributed solely to its taste but its high potassium content. To those people who do not have regular access to bananas, particularly those living in the Western Hemisphere the fruit can be really expensive compared to the areas near the tropics where this herb thrives. But if you know this, you will not fall behind in knowing that apples, which is abundant in cold Western countries, is also an excellent source of potassium. Here comes a substance made of apples that can give the daily potassium requirement of the body anytime of the day. Apple cider vinegar contains high levels of potassium, which controls sodium levels in the body. Sodium is associated with water retention, so getting rid of the excess is likely to result in weight loss. Nowadays, the common problem with many of our modern food choices is the increased amount of salt in many food preparations thus the effect of following a diet with more sodium content and less potassium. A deficiency in the proper amount of potassium that must be present in the body is undoubtedly one of the triggers of common bodily issues such as muscle weakness, fatigue, and cramps, to name a few. In addition, many experts attribute premature aging to a deficiency and potassium couple with an unhealthy lifestyle. So if looking and feeling older for your age is a regular experience, why not start consuming with your diet, food or supplements that are excellent sources of potassium. Keeping that in mind, adding ACV to your diet can help alleviate the risks of potassium deficiency symptoms earlier mentioned. In addition thereto, the consumption of potassium-rich ACV as a supplement, can also lower the risk of stroke and help prevent heart diseases.

Apple cider vinegar boosts the body's metabolism

If you are familiar with advertisements and commercials on the television promoting wellness and weight loss, you will often hear about the term metabolism. The fitness gurus and trainers always emphasized that a healthy metabolism is the key to effective weight loss without explaining how and why it is of such significance. But what is metabolism and how will it affect your goals of maintaining the ideal body mass? Metabolism is the process of energy production by converting the food or beverages we consume. In short, whatever we take in will be utilized by the body to support its energy needs. So it is necessary to be conscious of the quality of food we consume. That is why employing a diet technique accompanied by an exercise routine requires us to eat stuff the stuff that will supply the needed energy requirements. Apple cider vinegar revs up your body's metabolism by boosting digestion. As you know, a quicker metabolism means that you burn more calories, and it only takes a small quantity of ACV to start taking off the pounds with greater ease. No other sacrifice or effort is required! You may try other diet regimens which are claimed to improve your metabolism but you may not be aware that instead of helping out these may instead compromise the state of your metabolism. At this point the failure of the diet is attributable to the deprivation of nutrients by shying away from the food that may in fact be what your body actually needs for energy. You'll even notice a worsened effect on the body if your metabolism is unusually sluggish because you've been on a diet with no solid foods for a certain period of time. Thus the use of apple cider vinegar will improve your digestive processes without wreaking havoc on what constitutes as your normal eating habits. With ACV combined with a healthy and balanced selection of food plus exercise, weight loss is undoubtedly the end result. Aside from the benefit of improved digestion, toxins and wastes can be effectively excreted from the body.

Apple cider vinegar is rich in acetic acid

Another way in which ACV boosts your metabolism is due to its main component, acetic acid, which when mixed with food increases absorption of proteins by the body. Acetic acid in ACV may account for that unbearable smell distinct to this type of vinegar but it is a key composition of ACV that benefits the body in more ways that you can think of like maintaining an ideal body weight. The acetic acid in ACV forces the body to use more oxygen, resulting in a drastic increase in metabolic rate of which effect leads to your body burning about thrice as many calories as usual—regardless of whether you're engaging in strenuous physical exercise, resting, or simply going about your normal activities. You can forget about starving yourself of the food like some diet programs advise you to do. Who doesn't want to eat normally, right? Worry not by taking the apple cider vinegar as a supplement and satisfy your cravings with food that will surely sustain your body and satisfy those cravings. Of course, the more calories you burn, the more pounds you lose!

Cure for irritable bowel syndrome

Have you been feeling too stressed or depressed lately that it is affecting your daily bathroom routine? Yours may be a case of a disorder called an irritable bowel syndrome (IBS) which commonly affects the colon or what we call the large intestine. For better understanding of your symptoms a visit to a general practitioner may enlighten you about how to deal with it through medical advice and possible prescription. Although some sufferers of IBS may show severe symptoms like diarrhea, bloating, gassy stomach and cramping-conditions which need to be managed for some time, there are easy and self-aid remedies known to be safe and effective to comfort IBS sufferers. For natural alternatives then you need not look beyond the kitchen's pantry. All that you may possibly need is a dose of ACV. Apple cider vinegar's beneficial properties can achieve the normal and healthy digestion process which helps prevent the instances of diarrhea and irritable bowel syndrome. This allows the body to effectively neutralize the nutrients from the food you eat. At the same time, ACV helps the intestinal walls to push out unwanted fats so they aren't absorb and stored in the body, thus preventing weight gain.

Apple cider vinegar is rich in tryptophan

Tryptophan is one of the amino acids that are released when proteins are digested. Tryptophan stimulates the body to produce serotonin, which is very effective in relaxing the mind and in curbing emotional eating (stress-related eating).No wonder depressed and stressed people seek comfort food to release tension because we crave the neurotransmitter serotonin necessary to elevate our mood. When you were younger, you may have been told that taking a glass of milk will help you sleep soundly. That is because milk contains tryptophan to help you relax. But if you are someone who has a love and hate relationship with milk and other dairy products due to lactose intolerance, but is in search of the calming properties of a glass of milk before bedtime to cure your i insomnia, then a glass of warm water with a teaspoon of ACV before sleeping is a nice alternative. An additional benefit is burning of unwanted calories to reduce weight while you sleep.

Alkaline acid balance

According to experts the normal pH level of the body is 7.30 to 7.45. A pH level well within the normal range is slightly alkaline. You may either be on the alkaline or acidic side of the pH scale. If you want to maintain the normal pH level of the body you must attain the ideal pH level. This is relevant and of great significance due to its critical relationship with what constitutes a healthy body. A good, normal pH level will shield you from getting acquiring various diseases and ailments. It is common knowledge that the vinegar is an acidic substance however it provides an amazingly alkaline effect to the body creating a balance between what is basic and acidic. Another excellent feature of ACV is its ability to make our pH level move to the more alkaline scale despite being acidic. The body with a normal pH level can also cure itself effectively against infections and transforms toxins to a less toxic version of themselves lessening their harmful impact to our health. Taking two tablespoons of apple cider vinegar every day maintains the recommended (healthy) pH level in the body. This can give you more energy, which lets you exercise harder, which in turn lets you lose weight more quickly and easily.

Note: In losing weight, it is understandable that you want quick and visible results in the shortest time possible. But this is not actually the realistic and healthy way of reducing the unwanted fats in the body. If you are obese, losing 15 pounds may seem like nothing, and you may feel that trying ACV would be a waste of your time. But how often do you find an effective weight loss technique with so few rules about what you can and can't do? To be sure, if you want to lose a lot of weight you should combine ACV with various lifestyle changes. For instance, you could also reduce or eliminate excess sugar and bad fat and consume more veggies, water and fruits. Physical exercise is also important in losing unwanted fat. With any luck, ACV could be the little push that gets you started on a multitude of healthier habits!

DETOXIFICATION

Apple cider vinegar is also widely used for detoxifying the body. Unfortunately, in today's world there are health-damaging toxins all around us—in the air we breathe, the water we drink and the food we eat. Despite the conscious efforts on our part to live healthily, it is still a wise choice to assist the body in eliminating waste. Thus, regular detoxification is a necessity if we are to achieve an optimal quality of life. In simple terms, detoxification is the process of flushing toxins from the body. With a proper detox you can expect to regain your body's status quo. There are numerous detoxification techniques exist, but a lot of them are pretty extreme. Are you interested in going on a 45-day juice fast? I didn't think so. Apple cider vinegar is one of the easiest and most natural ways of detoxifying the body, as well as one of the safest. If you opt for ACV for detoxification, you will be taking a natural remedy that is rich in vitamins, natural enzymes, and minerals and has zero side effects. You won't have to worry about depriving your body of essential nutrients. No other detoxification technique provides all of that.

Certain components of ACV dissolve mucus and cleanse the lymph nodes, which improves lymph circulation. The accumulation of mucus and phlegm in the respiratory tract blocks the airway passages making it difficult to breathe for an individual. The lymphatic system works closely with the immune system to shield the body from disease-causing organisms and infections. A healthier lymphatic system is usually more effective in dealing with mucus congestion, sinus infections, and allergies. ACV also binds to many of the toxins that accumulate in the body, which makes it easier for the body to eliminate them and helps improve immune system response. Additionally, taking ACV daily improves digestion and general gastric health, and the better the body digests food, the faster it is to absorb the nutrients and remove any toxins before they can accumulate to harmful levels.

If you want to get the best results, it is wise to go for the best product, and with ACV you should opt for the raw, unprocessed, unfiltered and unpasteurized form with the "mother" in it. The organically produced ACV is the best option because you can avoid the chemical additives and artificial flavors mixed with some products to make the vinegar tasty. Some of the available choices of ACV which can be found in your local grocery aisles that appear clean and well-filtered are in fact the well-processed ones which are marketed to be promising but the manner of manufacture have already altered the beneficial aspects of the really healthful apple cider. The choice of low quality apple cider brands, which turned out to be processed/pasteurized vinegar only will bring forth unsatisfactory results that are far less than you expected. Make sure you're not cheated by the cheap imitations of apple cider vinegar; these are actually just white distilled vinegar with some caramel coloring added. If you want to be sure of your ACV, you may actually want to make it yourself from scraps or whole apples. You'll find detailed instructions later in the book.

For detoxification purposes, take at least one to three tablespoons of ACV in a glass of water before your meals to make the most of its effect of aiding digestion. That amount will ensure substantial results, but you may also want to use ACV as an ingredient in your meals for more complete elimination of toxins. For best results, you should use ACV in combination with a natural, healthy lifestyle. Here are some practices you may want to adopt:

#1: Reduce your exposure to toxins by using natural beauty products and household cleansers. There are always effective and organic alternatives.

#2: Look for ways of incorporating more uncooked (raw) foods in your diet, as these have essential enzymes that facilitate the detoxification process. In some instances over-exposure of the foods to heat during the cooking process lowers the level of nutrients in the food.

#3: Start drinking more filtered water to minimize your exposure to toxins. Almost all of our bodily processes depend on water. Drinking more pure water also causes your body to go through a natural detoxification process. Lastly, let us not forget about hydration as water keeps most of our organs, particularly the skin, and the largest organ of the body in tip-top condition.

#4: Eat more organic foods to reduce your exposure to toxins. You should also start reducing your consumption of processed foods, even when they are labeled organic.

#5: Eat a balanced diet composed of unprocessed natural ingredients to provide the nutrients your body needs to purify itself. There is nothing better than allowing your body to cleanse on its own by sustaining it with good fuel-nutritious and healthy food that is!

#6: Engage in plenty of physical exercise to enhance the functioning of the lymphatic and circulatory systems, as these are very important in full body detoxification. Remember, bodily activities will make you physically fit and improve your total health inside and out.

Here are a couple of ways to use ACV for detoxification that guarantee good results:

ACV detox bath

How in the world is a bath related to detox, you might say? Taking a bath may just be a very common activity for most of us and nothing makes it any special than allowing the outer body to feel refreshed by removing all the grime, germs as well as odor that clung to the skin on a day-to-day basis. But putting bathing to a notch higher than what we normally consider it, a bath is the perfect opportunity to eliminate wastes from in and out of the body. It is not only a matter of cleansing you're the external body but also the internal regions. While you take a bath, you sweat to excrete the wastes through your skin. Make use of a detox bath to help rid the body of harmful toxins; reduce the tensions in the mind, and provide that support needed to support the optimal functions of the various systems of the body. They're using ACV in detox bath to comfort conditions like arthritis, gout, and anything else caused by inflammation. This is a great bath to take if you need to sweat out the toxins and if you also want to be certain that you get to sleep without lying awake with a drifting mind.

You can take a hot bath prepared using a cup of Epsom salts and a cup of vinegar to draw toxins out of your skin. You have to soak in the mixture for 20-30 minutes to rid your skin of toxins. This is a good bath to take if you feel you need to sweat the toxins out, and also if you want to make sure that you get to sleep without lying awake with a wandering mind. This mixture is also very helpful in relieving joint pain and other skin conditions such as acne and eczema.

ACV Detox Tea Drink

Ingredients

- 2 tablespoons of lemon juice

- 2 tablespoons of ACV

- 1 teaspoon of cinnamon

- 12 ounces of filtered water at room temperature

- A dash of cayenne pepper

- Stevia powder to taste

Directions

1. Mix the ingredients in a glass, shake thoroughly, and then consume immediately.

2. For best results, take the mixture at least three times a day.

3. Soaking can help you to soften the taste of apple cider vinegar.

CHAPTER 3:
USING APPLE CIDER VINEGAR TO STAY HEALTHY

Apple cider vinegar can help with everything from minor health problems to complicated and potentially fatal medical condition. The prospective application of this substance for many medical ailments has been known for ages since the time of the renowned doctor, Hippocrates, who himself advocated the use of vinegar for the treatment of his own patients. It makes one wonder why physicians never advice to include supplementation of apple cider vinegar to enhance the effect of the medications they prescribe to their clients. Such reputation of the apple cider vinegar when it comes to healing the body will lead you to the conclusion that apple cider promotes the overall wellness of those who use it. Many of ACV's proponents believe that this is because its high concentration of acetic acid increases the body's ability to absorb vitamins and minerals from foods. In fact, that's far from the only good thing about ACV: it also contains potassium, enzymes, and other organic acids such as lactic acid and propionic acid. These will make you feel better and confer a host of health benefits if you drink ACV regularly.

To control blood sugar

Apple cider vinegar appears to have a comparable effect as insulin-controlling medications like acarbose and metformin. In effect, both the acarbose and metformin are prescribed to treat people with Type 2 diabetes and are usually combined with insulin and other diabetes medications to ensure efficacy. Since general practitioners advice these medicines to patients the drugs are the only popular means of helping diabetes sufferers. Patients are often limited to other recourses such as alternative medicines or herbal medications to control the state and progression of their disease. Despite being written in prescriptions to diabetes sufferers, said medicines often prescribed by GPs to patients with blood sugar problems are under fire recently due to reported side effects like bladder and heart complications. This is the risks often associated with prescribed medicines because side effects may be present to complicate further an existing medical condition. To avoid further risks to their health and perhaps to save on costs, people are reaching out to safer alternatives like apple cider vinegar. In fact studies have revealed that doses of ACV before meals and bedtime can assist in the management of blood glucose levels. It is even more amazing to know that the vinegar has properties that possess the combined efficacy of several diabetes drugs at a fraction of the cost. How? ACV slows the absorption of carbohydrates in the blood as is the starch to sugar. Diabetics who use ACV consistently often experience significant decreases in blood sugar, although this effect has not been fully proven by scientists. But numerous studies suggest that any kind of vinegar can be very effective in fighting diabetes. A study performed at Arizona State University found out that apple cider vinegar slows the rate blood sugar levels rise after a meal. In one, people who consumed at least two tablespoons of ACV just before bedtime experienced favorable changes in blood sugar and glucose levels the following day.

To lower cholesterol levels

The negative effects of high level of cholesterol to the body are well-documented by many studies. Cholesterol is needed at some point by the body to function but it should not be at an amount that the body can no longer utilize. Although there are good and bad cholesterol from various sources, you must to stay away from the harmful ones that promote many diseases that are known to man. A lot of people who are found to have a high cholesterol levels in their body are also observed to be suffering from obesity and blood pressure issues. Perhaps due to the consumption of unhealthy food and the lack of physical exercise, the amount of cholesterol in the blood can elevate to an alarming level. Foods which contains a lot of bad cholesterol are often described to be oily, processed, salty and sadly, delicious. Consuming these on a regular basis can result to too much cholesterol and consequently weight gain. A high cholesterol level will interfere with the proper flow of blood in the body thus exposing you to various diseases like heart problems, diabetes, kidney complications and many others. Acidic and sour substances can help ease cholesterol but care must be taken because some acids also interfere with the normal digestive processes. It is perfect to find an acid that can neutralize fats and cholesterol but will not have a drastic consequence to your stomach. Try apple cider vinegar in appropriate doses. To combat and at least minimize the effects of cholesterol, supplementation of apple cider vinegar with your regular diet is never a bad idea. The high levels of acetic acid and potassium in ACV are known to lower bad cholesterol levels. These components cause the blood to become thinner, thus allowing it to circulate with greater ease. Cholesterol level scan drop significantly after as little as a month of daily ACV use.

To relieve joint pain and arthritis

Excessive accumulation of toxin crystals in combination with mineral deficiency is a major contributing factor for arthritis and many other diseases associated with joint stiffness. Often it is the elderly and people with auto-immune disorders that are often plagued with such issues. Arthritis and joint pain sufferers are slowed in terms of mobility that prevents them from engaging in their normal daily routines. If you are one to suffer from arthritis it is not to your advantage to bear the pain and continuously rely on medications. It is known that arthritis is a chronic medical issue for individuals whose tissues suffer degeneration causing them the characteristic stiffness and inflammation which is symptomatic of arthritis sufferers. There is no need to suffer in silence because you can try something that poses little risk if you also happen to be taking other medications. What you need is a good supplement in the form of apple cider vinegar. The high phosphorous, magnesium, calcium and potassium content of ACV acts to prevent excessive buildup of toxin crystals in the joints. And as we learned in the previous chapter, ACV has potent detoxification properties because it binds to toxins and allows them to be flushed out of the body before they can accumulate to toxic levels in the joints. Drinking ACV is very effective for this purpose, relieving the muscles and joints from severe pain brought about by the inflammation. But to ensure the efficacy of apple cider vinegar, you should also apply it directly on the affected joint to relieve pain and stiffness. Just mix two tablespoons of apple cider vinegar with one tablespoon of organic virgin coconut oil and then massage over the affected area. It also helps to soak your hands or feet for several minutes in about six cups of warm water mixed with one cup of ACV to reduce pain.

To relieve pain from insect stings and bites

Who doesn't love being outdoors? It's always a breath of fresh air to experience nature outside the comforts of our home. However being one with Mother Nature has its price. It is not uncommon to get bitten or stung by organisms while taking a walk in the park or lying down in the grass. Notice a red, itchy and swelling bump in your skin? You might have just been bitten by an insect. You are aware that the first thing you should do is apply first aid treatment to the affected area. No need to run to the medicine cabinet and grab the good old insect bite salve. Instead there is a nice kitchen alternative, used by a few, who knew of the good natural and alternatives that are effective and chemical-free. If you have apple cider vinegar bottle ion the kitchen, it's time to put it to some other good use than just being your average condiment. Just take some apple cider vinegar and rub some of it to soothe the pain or itchiness and to control the swelling of the insect bite. So next time you're stung by a bee or any other insect, ACV is the easiest way to relieve the pain—just apply it to the sting to get the needed relief.

As a remedy for fatigue and exhaustion

In your day-to-day life the unexpected lack of energy and weariness can stop you from finishing all your daily tasks. When you engage in strenuous physical exercise, the levels of stress in your body rise, making you feel exhausted. This is just the normal aftermath of engaging in work and activity because you burned energy. However for some people, they may feel exhausted and constantly tired despite not doing anything. This is not enough to conclude that they are lazy but they are probably suffering from what experts call as chronic fatigue. Chronic fatigue is not your ordinary fatigue because this is persistent and may continue for a long period of time for no reasonable causes or underlying medical issue. It is surprising but this is not also a psychological issue because it is a means of the body to call your attention to its present state. You may have deprived your body of the needed sleep, proper diet and exercise so there is the accumulation of tension in the body which must be released. It is best to let the body recuperate and what better alternative to let the body heal itself by taking apple cider vinegar doses. To combat weakness apple cider vinegar can help the body produce the needed energy to start and end your day. Although ACV contains a lot of acetic acid, it also has potassium and various enzymes that prevent acetic acid from building up in the body. That means you can use ACV as an energy drink to guarantee a smooth workout! All you have to do is add ACV to a glass of chilled carrot or tomato juice to unlock its full power. Take some rest while you enjoy your favorite beverage mixed with apple cider vinegar goodness.

As an immune system booster

It is already cliché to hear the saying "An apple a day keeps the doctor away."But despite repetition the truth about this saying will never pass because apples can be the key to avoid your body from getting sick every time. It is first important to get reacquainted with what the immune system can do for us. The immune system is the body's defense against bacteria, viruses and other disease-causing microorganisms that at anytime may enter the body. Constantly, we are bombarded by these elements and the immune system continuously works all the time while the body functions. So it will be highly beneficial to the body if you will eat fruits and vegetables, known to fuel and sustain the body. Apples are always good additions to your diet. If not apple, you can use its derivative, the apple cider vinegar. Apple cider vinegar contains malic acid, which is an antiviral, antifungal and antibacterial agent that is effective in preventing fever and colds, as well as alleviating various allergies. Malic acid is naturally present in many types of fruits and vegetables that humans consume, particularly apples. In the human body, when carbohydrates are converted into energy malic acid is the end product. The significance of malic acid lies in the fact that it facilitates the activation of the immune system to react to any foreign elements that can make the body sick. Therefore, the consumption of apple cider vinegar benefits the body to take advantage of a wide range of essential minerals and trace elements like calcium, potassium, chlorine, magnesium, copper, silicon, iron, sodium, phosphorous and fluorine, which are all essential for maintaining a healthy immune system.

As a remedy for food poisoning

The cases of victims of food borne illnesses on the rise are well-documented by many media outlets causing concern among the populace. There are many factors that may cause the frequency of such incidents and corollary thereto, we should gain a better understanding of how we can pinpoint and avoid getting sick by contaminated food and water. Food borne illnesses are caused by consuming contaminated food items where bacteria, parasites or viruses thrive. Also known as food poisoning, this is a possible result of mishandling or inadequate food preparations. If suffering from the same, a person may feel nausea, abdominal cramps, vomiting, weakness, diarrhea and severe dehydration. Such affliction is not something that one can easily deal with. After knowing how we can acquire such a disease it is also good to know and apply preventive measures to make help the body cope with food poisoning symptoms. Just take note however that it is still best to bring a suspected patient to the hospital if there are symptoms of food poisoning for immediate medical treatment. If in cases that the symptoms are mild and will not entail hospitalization, the acidity of ACV can kill bacteria that caused the sickness as an immediate relief. To make it more effective for this purpose, drink it more concentrated than usual (this doesn't mean you shouldn't dilute it a little!), and be sure to take it when your stomach is empty.

As a remedy for nasal congestion

With the arrival of the cold season the possibility of catching any of the numerous strains of the cold virus is inevitable unless you have an ironclad immune system. Other than colds, the flu and other allergic reactions may also trigger a nasal congestion. Nothing irritates cold sufferers more than a stuffy nose caused by the swelling of the nasal passages and accumulation of mucus. This condition leads to difficulty in breathing. Without immediate treatment, a congested nasal cavity can worsen and result to problems like ear infection, lack of sleep, among others. It is not wise to just leave a stuffy nose be. You yourself can remedy your situation and reduce the discomfort by trying alternative and simple remedies. Do not simply reach out for that nasal decongestant which has side effects. If you need to avoid the drowsy effect but would like immediate relief to that stuffy nose, there several things you can try at home. There are numerous ways to clear a decongested nose. In addition to trying out the favorite chicken noodle soup to cure your colds, the use of apple cider vinegar can quickly clear that blocked nose of yours.ACV has the ability to thin mucus, and the potassium and acetic acid it contains prevent the accumulation of bacteria within the sinus, making it ideal for decongesting a stuffy nose. To use ACV to cure nasal congestion, mix a tablespoon of it in a glass of warm water. You may add a tablespoon of honey if desired. This concoction can be consumed up to two or three times a day for several days until the stuffy nose is relieved.

As a remedy for indigestion

Don't you just love to eat like I do? I guess you know that we have been constantly told that moderation is key to almost everything, especially our diets but it just difficult to restrain yourself from taking the second or so helping of your favorite dish. It is such an agony to stop thy self, right? And indeed in the end you may even regret your choice of eating too much. Why so? Because what comes next is something that most people would never wish to experience. Indigestion. Although it is not always a serious problem unless it is accompanied by several other symptoms. Some foods are so tasty that you would eat them till you dropped if it weren't for the indigestion and other problems involved in overeating. Indigestion is described as a feeling of discomfort in the upper part of the abdominal cavity or the unexpected feeling of fullness despite consuming a small portion of food. If you're going to a buffet or planning to indulge in your favorite food or dish, try drinking a mix of ACV (1 tablespoon) and honey (1 tablespoon) in about 8 ounces of water 20-30 minutes before your meal to minimize the possibility of having an upset stomach should you overeat. This can be quite effective in preventing other issues related to indigestion such as stomach cramps, nausea, heartburn, and acid reflux that you might otherwise experience. Should your indigestion persists it's wise to consult your physician

As a sore throat remedy

Apple cider vinegar is not a total replacement for medications prescribed by your doctor in case you have a painful sore throat. If you have a persisting pain, itchiness, dryness and swelling in your throat it's an advisable remedy to gargle a mixture of water and ACV. Since it is a substance that has a strong acidic property it can be an effective remedy to combat sore throats due to colds or even an infection due to the bacteria *streptococcus*, otherwise known as a "Strep Throat". The bacteria that cause sore throat are sensitive to acidity, and you can balance the body's pH to make it harder for them to grow by gargling a quarter cup of apple cider vinegar mixed with water. Do this every hour when you feel like you're coming down with a sore throat and you'll soon experience the needed relief.

As a remedy for hiccups

There are sudden involuntary contractions of the muscles of the diaphragm while the voice box contracts. This creates that mildly bothersome hiccup which may have been caused by drinking or eating too fast. Hiccups may go away on its own but you can shorten the length of your hiccups by easing the irritation in the diaphragm by using apple cider vinegar. The use of ACV helps restores diaphragm spasms and improves the elimination of stomach acids. Taking a teaspoon of apple cider vinegar can put a quick end to hiccups because the sour taste of ACV usually overwhelms the nerves in the mouth, making them relax and effectively ending the annoying phenomenon.

As a remedy for leg cramps

The feeling of a sudden tightening and pain in the legs, also known as muscle cramps occurring on the leg is not a nice experience. This condition may be a result of over-exerted muscles due to heavy exercise, nutrient deficiency and even lack of hydration. Leg cramps are usually harmless and can be a common experience but it is a likely evidence of inadequate potassium levels in the body, and you can probably guess what that means. To lessen the incidence of leg cramps it can help to drink a solution with apple cider on a regular basis. Yes, apple cider vinegar or ACV is rich in potassium, so taking it can be effective in ending leg cramps. For instant relief, just drink a mixture of two tablespoons of apple cider vinegar, one tablespoon of honey and eight ounces of water.

To relieve asthma

Based on Statistics, asthma is a lung condition that affects around 34 million of people in the United States alone. It is characterized by inflammation of the airway passages that results to difficulty in breathing, coughing and to some extent wheezing. To suffer from this condition, it is a relatable experience to have an extreme difficulty in taking in air. In many cases asthma is triggered by specific stimuli like dusts, smoke or exhaustion that can be a real nuisance to some since it interferes with the ordinary activities and may even be life threatening to others. There are ways where ACV assists asthma sufferers. Although patients rely on inhalers and spray medications, apple cider vinegar may provide a natural and alternative relief. When you drink a glass of water mixed with a tablespoon of apple cider vinegar, you are likely to experience improved breathing. ACV relaxes the throat muscles, which in turn makes it easier to breathe, even during an asthma attack. However, it shouldn't be used as a complete substitute for your asthma medication or spray.

To relieve stomach woes

There are a lot of instances where we can suffer an upset stomach. It is one of the most uncomfortable feelings in the body. If you suffer from spasms, diarrhea or any other stomach problems, you may avoid reaching out for the medicine cabinet because apple cider vinegar could be the cure you've been looking for rather than immediate recourse to pharmaceutical remedies which may have adverse side effects. Drinking at least two tablespoons of ACV mixed with water or clear juices should end your problems.

As a perfect defense mechanism against CANDIDA (yeast overgrowth)

As you know by now, apple cider vinegar is acidic in nature. Yeast doesn't grow well in acidic environments, so taking ACV helps prevent excessive accumulation of yeast in the body. An excessive accumulation of yeast can have a negative impact to the skin, mouth, throat, genitals and blood. Said body parts already have small portions of these fungal growth but any abnormal increase may result to infection. Therefore apple cider vinegar with its acidic properties can control the overgrowth of yeast by eliminating sugar, which is the food source of yeasts and fungi. (Aside from its acidity, ACV also has enzymes that combat yeast.) A tablespoon of ACV each day is enough, but it may not work immediately. Don't be scared if your yeast problem seems to be getting worse at first; just continue taking ACV and you'll start feeling better soon. Soaking in a tub of warm water mixed with 1.5 cups of ACV for 20 minutes is also very effective in getting rid of yeast infections.

As a remedy for bad breath

It can be both embarrassing and frustrating to have bad breath. Bad breath is medically known as "halitosis". It may be attributed to poor dental hygiene or an underlying medical issue like an infection somewhere in the body. So if you wonder why you cannot still gain that fresh breath even if you have the best oral hygiene habits, (regular brushing and dental checkups) you can try apple cider vinegar. Also thanks to its acidity, apple cider vinegar has antiseptic properties that make it an ideal remedy for halitosis or bad breath. The acid breaks down plaque and bacteria that cause bad breath. As halitosis may also be a consequence of a faulty digestive system or indigestion, using apple cider as a supplement may aid in proper digestion thus clearing the dilemma. Lastly, the nutrients and minerals present in ACV are beneficial to maintain healthy teeth and gums. To gain the benefits just add a tablespoon of apple cider vinegar to a cup of water, gargle the mixture for about 15 seconds, and then spit the solution out. Repeat until the cup is empty. We hope you can use apple cider vinegar if you have such issues but remember to dilute ACV properly since a strong concoction may damage the enamel of your teeth.

As a remedy for body odor

As part of proper hygiene, maintaining a clean body is a must. Cleanliness however is not only about looking good and neat, but also about smelling fresh and divine. It will not be helpful to bathe in perfume to mask an existing body odor. Because instead of reducing the smell it will exacerbate the problem. The common cause of body odor is often associated with improper bodily hygiene, underlying medical condition, food choices, overactive sweat glands and some other possible conditions. If you feel that the commercial deodorants are not that effective or incompatible with your condition, try out some alternatives like apple cider vinegar. You do not need to worry about sticking out due to the sour scent like a salad's vinaigrette. You would be surprised that despite the strong smell of apple cider vinegar, its application will prevent the stinky body odor sans the distinct scent. Indeed, there is no need to fret about the permanent smell of vinegar because once it is applied; the apple cider smell will soon dissipate. But the effect will be an improvement in the scent of the body since it has the ability to neutralize odor-causing bacteria. We already learned that apple cider vinegar helps balance your internal pH. It can also adjust the pH of your skin, which in turn helps to fight off bacteria that cause unpleasant body odor. You can do this at least once a week after bathing. You can use apple cider vinegar instead of your regular underarm deodorant; just wipe your armpits once every morning with undiluted ACV. The unpleasant smell of the feet is also annoying and may cause loss of confidence whenever you take off your socks or footwear. But there is no bad smell that apple cider vinegar cannot remedy. For foot odor, dilute 1/3 cup of ACV in warm water and soak your feet in the mixture for up to 15 minutes once every week. If you find this effective, you may even swap your commercial deodorant for this organic remedy at a cheaper price!

As a cure for UTI (urinary tract infections)

The affliction of Urinary Tract Infection is no easy business. It can be both painful and embarrassing because the experience of urinating-as a way to excrete wastes through urine is accompanied by a burning sensation and a back or stomach pain. This condition can be more common to women than men such that the existence of the condition is often brushed aside as a symptom of the menstrual cycle. There may be a lot of possible causes for UTI but the biggest concern is providing relief to treat and prevent further difficulties. Since apple cider vinegar can work as an antibiotic to the effect of lessening complications of the infection it is a perfect alternative remedy. The potassium and different active enzymes in ACV are very effective in combating the bacteria that cause UTI. If you suffer from this condition, drink a glass of water mixed with two tablespoons of ACV twice a day for several days; you can add lemon juice and honey to sweeten it. You can also add a few drops of ACV to your bath water to relieve the burning sensation that often accompanies UTI.

As a growth hormone production boost

If you want your kids to grow faster and taller, apple cider vinegar could be your secret weapon. Parents think that they can rely on growth enhancing supplements and vitamins that often come with a hefty price tag to help their kids grow taller at a faster rate. However there are negative effects of using growth hormones in children's supplements. The controversy surrounding growth hormones are still being subject of debates but several independent studies in the past reveal scary side effects. Some of these effects like leukemia, abnormal or decreased sensations in several parts of the body, blurred vision, and abnormal heart beat are closely linked to administering growth hormone supplements to children at a young age. We know that it is never good to go beyond what genetics can offer to alter the appearance and height of our children. So to be safe parents must be aware of these complications and may instead look towards alternative substances that can help promote growth naturally. Substances that encourage growth by facilitating cell repair and reproduction can be found in apple cider vinegar. It has enzymes and nutrients that are very effective in helping your body break down the proteins that you eat into amino acids. The increased availability of amino acids allows the body to produce more growth hormone. (As an added benefit, your body breaks down more fat when more growth hormone is present. This is another reason that ACV is so effective in helping you maintain or lose weight.) To increase production of growth hormone, mix one or two tablespoons of ACV in water and drink before every meal.

CHAPTER 4:
USE APPLE CIDER VINEGAR FOR BEAUTIFUL SKIN

It is a common dictum that beauty is skin deep, yet we know that the present era has its own standard of what it considers as beautiful. Despite changing trends in this aspect, one of the things that remained constant is the appreciation for beautiful and perfect skin. As the largest organ of the body, the skin is one of the indicators of good health. Most possibly due to many efforts of transforming skin to its most beautiful state, it is one of the parts of our body prone to abuse and deterioration. With many cosmetic products to choose from nowadays that claim to improve the skin, there is a tendency to over-expose the organ to harsh chemicals that do more harm than good. Some of these chemicals can be found in whitening agents, firming lotions, make-up, hair removal creams and other near-absurd products that promote extreme and unrealistic expectations of beauty. With many people suffering from cancers and diseases that are now being linked to beauty treatments it is not surprising that some would like to ditch their chemically-laden beauty products and substitute with natural and organic beauty hacks. Alongside the movement to choose a natural approach to beauty it's high time to introduce the beautifying benefits of apple cider vinegar to the skin. I know it sounds weird to apply something that you would ordinarily eat on your skin. However, apple cider vinegar or ACV is one of those exceptional items that can serve all purposes; you can drink it, soak your body in it, or apply it on your skin to achieve different miraculous results! The strong smell of ACV may make you skeptical about slathering it on your skin, but many people do so anyway, so it's not hard to guess that ACV has unique properties that may it worthwhile. What are they? Regular users of ACV say that it has the power to heal and improve the skin's condition. ACV is believed to enhance blood circulation within the small capillaries in the skin. It also has antiseptic properties that cure and prevent bacterial skin infections like acne. As already mentioned, ACV's acetic acid content can help to balance skin pH levels. This in turn helps prevent and lessen acne breakouts, skin peeling, skin scaling, and excessive oil production. ACV normalizes sebum production, ensuring that the skin is not too dry or too oily. It also contains hydroxyl acids, which are very effective in getting rid of dead skin cells, giving your skin a healthier, younger look.

IN EVERYDAY SKIN CARE

Apple cider vinegar has a wide range of skincare applications and a wide range of benefits. As a phase in taking care of your skin, the aspect of skincare should not be taken for granted because this stage will prepare the skin by using beneficial products such as the apple cider vinegar. This section will discuss practical ways you can use it every day to attain the beautiful look you've been longing for. You'll learn the steps for using apple cider vinegar in different situations to cure various skin problems.

As a facial wash

The use of an effective facial wash or cleanser as the basic step in your beauty regimen will help against breakouts and clear skin blemishes. There are so many facial wash brands made available commercially and can be bought form the pharmacy and the supermarket that will suit your very skin needs. However even you if you will try a multitude of products you just cannot get the perfect product for the needs of your skin.

If you are still in search for that wonderful cleanser then perhaps apple cider vinegar is perfect for you without the undesirable dryness, flaking and harsh chemicals that other commercial face washes can offer. To this effect apple cider vinegar can also double as a gentle and organic face cleanser. Mix about 2 tablespoons of apple cider vinegar with 6 tablespoons of warm water (10 tablespoons if you have sensitive skin).Wash your face with warm water, then dip a cotton ball into the mixture and apply it on your neck and face. Use a gentle upward motion and continue until the cotton ball is free of dirt.

Note: Even if you don't like the smell, do not wash off the ACV for at least 15 minutes. If the smell doesn't bother you, you can actually apply a moisturizer immediately; you don't have to wash it!

Mixed with herbs

Mixing apple cider vinegar with aromatic herbs like lavender, rosewood, and rosemary increases its potency. These herbs contain essential oils that are very effective in enhancing the skin's appearance and health. They also have excellent healing properties and can be mixed in quantities to adjust to skin conditions. When you use herbal apple cider vinegar, your skin will benefit by improving the suppleness and texture and gaining that youthful appearance that can hide signs of aging. So, how do you make herbal ACV? It is simple:

Method 1

Ingredients

- 3 ounces of elder flowers

- 2 pints of apple cider vinegar

- 2 ounces of calendula

Method 2

Ingredients

- 1 ounce of lavender

- Linden flowers

- 2 pints of apple cider vinegar

- Rose petals

Directions

Pour the apple cider vinegar into a jar, add the plant materials, secure the lid tightly and place in a warm place. Let the plant materials macerate for up to 2 weeks, then strain and store the contents in a clean bottle.

How to use it

For a facial wash, dissolve 1 tablespoon of the mixture in a cup of spring water then wash your face.

For a full body bath, dissolve up to 5 tablespoons of the mixture in a tub filled with water. Here is another recipe using essential oils that makes an effective skincare concoction for home use:

Ingredients

- 3/5 teaspoons of lavender essential oil

- 1 cup of filtered water

- 2/5 teaspoons of rosewood essential oil

- 3/5 teaspoons of rosemary essential oil

- 2 tablespoons of glycerin

- 17.5 fluid ounce ACV

Directions

Mix all ingredients together then soak a ball of cotton in the mixture and dab all over your face. Let it dry before rinsing.

As a pH-balancing toner

If you can't face yourself in the mirror due to pimples and other skin problems, you may want to start using apple cider vinegar to ward off the pimple-causing bacteria. Pimples are clogged pores of our skin that became inflamed due to bacteria that entered the oil glands. Dirt may also cause pimples and if severe pimples can turn to acne. This skin condition should not be left untreated because if it worsens, permanent scarring may happen and cause damage the skin. If you cannot find a good product, try this kitchen alternative. Do this by a do-it-yourself toner made from apple cider vinegar. But do you actually need a toner in the first place? The answer is a resounding yes if you need a product to remove the remaining dirt and other particles that stayed even after washing your face. Other than that, an effective toner can help refine the appearance of your pores and control the production of sebum. That is the job of a good toner. What better alternative than to use than apple cider vinegar which has an excellent pH balance for your skin? Dissolving ½ cup of apple cider vinegar in 2 cups of distilled water could provide the cure for your condition. This concoction will unblock pores and remove dead skin cells that could be making your skin look less than its best.

Directions

Mix the ingredients and transfer to a sterilized glass bottle.

Use a clean cotton pad or ball to apply the toner to clean skin and leave it to dry before rinsing. You can then apply moisturizer immediately to keep the skin supple and looking healthy.

If you want to use it on the rest of your body to cure acne or other conditions, just place the mixture in a clean spray bottle and spray it on blackheads and back acne. It's a great way of keeping your skin healthy and youthful looking.

TIP: Shake well before use!

Detoxifying facemask

If you have acne and you can't use commercial cosmetic products because your skin seems too sensitive to them, apple cider vinegar could be your solution to the skin problem. A routine face mask may seem redundant and an unnecessary beauty step but it can help in more ways than one. By using a face mask, pamper yourself and your skin without spending so much right there and then, at the comforts of your home! IT'S better to use a natural and organic Do-it-yourself facemask with natural ingredients. You can use an apple cider vinegar blend to get rid of dirt located deep under your skin and even open up pores for a smoother, healthier and better looking complexion. With this concoction, you can get rid of rashes, pimples and many other annoying skin problems, leaving behind a smooth, pimple-free skin. So how do you make the concoction?

Ingredients

- 1 tablespoon of raw honey

- Apple cider vinegar (enough to soak a cotton ball)

- Bentonite clay

Directions

Mix equal parts of apple cider vinegar and bentonite clay then add honey and stir thoroughly until mixed well.

Apply the mixture on a clean face and let it sit for about 15 minutes before rinsing off with warm water.

PEPPER ROSE TONER

Does your skin feel itchy sometimes, or do you have an unusually oily face that makes you feel uncomfortable? If you haven't tried apple cider vinegar, please do! ACV mixed with rosemary essential oil and peppermint essential oil could be the cure you've been looking for. It will also help you brighten your skin in the process. It is the combined goodness of apple cider vinegar and rosemary in one!

Ingredients

- 10 drops of rosemary essential oil

- 2 tablespoons of apple cider vinegar

- 8 drops of peppermint essential oil

- 1 cup of distilled or filtered water

Directions

Combine the ingredients in a glass container and shake well before applying the concoction on your skin.

Apply the concoction on your skin daily.

Tip: You may want to reduce the apple cider vinegar to 1 tablespoon if you experience too much of a drying effect.

TO REDUCE AGE SPOTS

Got age spots? It is not an uncommon skin problem. Ideally this skin disorder will appear on people as part of the normal aging process or if they are always exposed to the sun's harmful ultraviolet rays. Also known as liver spots those individuals who have age spots can look older than their real age. If you are one who value clear and blemish-free skin then you can turn to apple cider vinegar to gradually remove the annoying spots. If you want a cheaper, natural and safe to use alternative apart from the commercially available beauty products, you may try apple cider vinegar toner instead of that expensive products in the market. It will reduce the appearance of consciously bothersome marks especially in your face. With apple cider vinegar or ACV you may not need to purchase those expensive products in the market:

Method 1 (apple cider vinegar mixed with orange juice)

Ingredients

- 1 tablespoon of orange juice

- 2 tablespoons of apple cider vinegar

Directions

Mix the ingredients thoroughly, soak a cotton pad or cotton ball in the mixture, then spot-treat the age spots.

Leave the treatment on overnight.

Tip: Follow the routine for 4-5 weeks for best results.

Method 2 (apple cider vinegar and onion juice)

Ingredients

- ¼ cup of apple cider vinegar

- ¼ cup of fresh onion juice (made from raw onion)

Directions

Mix the ingredients thoroughly, then apply the mixture on the age spots using a cotton swab; do this twice daily. Leave the treatment on overnight.

Tip: To avoid skin irritation, apply the mixture only on the age spots (not the surrounding areas of the skin). You may also want to put on some goggles if you are applying it on the face to avoid contact in the eyes.

TO RELIEVE SUNBURN

Summer is here and the heat is on! There are so many things that you can do under the blazing heat of the season but don't forget to protect yourself while you enjoy the sunshine. Although it's recommended that you avoid skin damage by exposing yourself to the sun for no more than 15 minutes at a time, that's not always possible when you're out and about. The sunburns that follow can make you feel sorry that you broke this rule, but you can neutralize them with apple cider vinegar. It relieves the pain and gets rid of the accompanying blistering and peeling of skin. Just add one cup of apple cider vinegar to warm bathwater and soak for about 8 minutes. Be prepared for an initial sting as the body gets used to the treatment!

TO BRIGHTEN SKIN

Exfoliation is one of the keys to having gorgeous skin. It is an important part of skin care that will benefit both the facial skin and body. The process of exfoliation removes the dead cells in the outermost layer of the skin while revealing that radiant skin beneath. In terms of frequency, proper exfoliation can be done once or twice a week to avoid skin damage. Using apple cider vinegar solution can also help you to exfoliate your skin. It provides a beautiful, natural glow that will make you confident about your looks. It also removes excess oil from the skin and reduces redness and swelling that is caused by acne. So how do you make it with apple cider vinegar and some other common yet effective ingredients?

Ingredients

- ½ ounce of apple cider vinegar

- 3 ounces of distilled water

- 5 plain, uncoated aspirin tablets

Directions

Mix the apple cider vinegar and the water in a bowl, and then use a mortar and pestle to crush the aspirin tablets into a fine powder. Add the powder to the ACV mixture and stir well until it is completely dissolved.

Apply this toner on your face weekly for several months until you start seeing results.

AS A MOISTURIZER

Got this itchy, dry, red or flaky skin? Then you're skin condition is probably in a state of dryness and that calls for a good measure of hydration. Dry skin should not be too bothersome but if you want great skin then it's time to start paying attention to providing it with a good amount of moisture. Hydration ensures that your skin is protected from free radicals and prevents unwanted aging. How do you keep your skin effectively hydrated? The habit of consuming enough water and fluids is one way. We often heard that a person should drink at least 8 glasses of water to fulfill the required amount that the body needs. However, this is disputed by some experts who believe that there is no hard and fast rule in the determination of the amount of water that a person should consume on a daily basis. The rule of 8 glasses forgets to take into account that we also get water from other sources like fruits and vegetables. So how will you determine the amount you need? Then always ensure that you drink water before and after meals and pay heed to the body's request to drink water each time despite your busy schedule. Dry and sensitive skin, will also benefit when using a good skin moisturizer. If you are looking for a natural and cheaper way to moisturize, you may take advantage of the moisturizing qualities of apple cider vinegar. Below is a recipe of how you can make a DIY apple cider vinegar moisturizer.

Ingredients

- 1 tablespoon of apple cider vinegar

- 3 drops of argan oil

- 4 tablespoons of green tea

Directions

Mix the ingredients in a bowl, and then transfer them to a spray bottle. Spray the mixture on your face whenever you need more moisture.

Tip: Shake well before use.

To remove warts

Got this pesky embarrassing thing called warts? They are usually harmless skin protrusions that appear on the top layer of the skin which they call epidermis. After some time, they may go away on their own or need to be treated to disappear from the skin. Still, after disappearing, some types of warts can recur after treatment. You know that warts appearing on parts of your body can be annoying and in some way embarrassing. And if you do want to get rid of them, try an effective apple cider vinegar recipe. Then try using this mixture of apple cider vinegar and garlic on the problem area:

Ingredients

- ½ clove of garlic

- ½ cup of apple cider vinegar (enough to soak a cotton bandage)

Directions

Crush the garlic and place it on the wart.

Soak a cotton bandage in ACV and use it to wrap the area with the wart. Leave it there overnight, remove the bandage in the morning, and then rinse the wart with cold water. Apply an adequate amount of castor oil on the wart, then cover the area with a dry bandage. Repeat this until the wart is completely cured.

To cure athlete's foot

Are you experiencing scaling, peeling, redness and blistering of your feet? Other than that, are there some noticeable skin growths in between your toes? If yes, then you may have developed athlete's foot since those earlier enumerated are the symptoms of the skin ailment. This condition is common and really contagious, affecting those individuals who often have sweaty feet or who were unfortunate in acquiring the fungal infection from someone through personal contact or through objects that are contaminated by infected individuals. In this situation, apple cider vinegar can help in curing athlete's foot. Do this by mixing equal parts of apple cider vinegar and water and applying the concoction to the affected area. This will put a stop to both the itching and the bad odor. If you want to make this mixture stronger and more effective, you can try adding Listerine mouthwash (the original variant).

To get rid of varicose veins

Do you have these blue, sometimes greenish, large and spidery veins on your legs? They may be the main reason why you do not like to wear shorts, skirts and dresses that can expose them. These abnormalities are actually the enlarged veins on the legs. They occur because of the increased pressures on the lower parts of the body due to walking upright and prolonged standing. Well, they are varicose veins and they can also be found in the feet. For some who think that varicose veins are minor cosmetic concerns, their issues may be a bit off to some who find the enlarged veins a reason for pain and discomfort. This is one of the reasons why some would search of means to alleviate the problem. Because varicose veins are actually a problem with the circulation of blood in the body, apple cider vinegar really helps for its ability to improve the function of the circulatory process. To get rid of varicose veins, place cotton or cloth soaked in apple cider vinegar on the swollen veins for up to 10 minutes, then massage your legs with strokes that move towards the heart.

For callus removal

Who doesn't want smooth hands and feet, right? When we exert effort to do some activities we cannot help but engage the skin and the muscles to perform various tasks. But this exposure to friction or pressure can harden some parts or layers of our skin making it more rough and thick in both feel and appearance than others. This should be regarded as a normal reaction of the skin and is no cause for concern. As an exception, some who have calluses can at be considered at risk because these can cause complications particularly with those who have diabetes. In general, calluses hardly need treatment, unless they cause you real discomfort. If you want them removed, here is a way to get rid of them naturally and without a need for an expensive cosmetic procedure. Just use this apple cider vinegar mixture! For the best results, soak your hands or feet in concentrated (undiluted) apple cider vinegar for 30-60 minutes, then use pumice stone to get rid of any toughened skin. Once you remove the skin, soak again for about 15 minutes and rinse. Repeat the process every week.

To cure other skin problems

Just earlier, ways of improving some skin issues using apple cider vinegar were discussed. In this next elaboration, more skin-friendly ways of utilizing the substance will be mentioned. This is just proof of endless possibilities of using apple cider to improve your skin's state. Apart from those already identified and explained, apple cider vinegar is also a good cleanser for the skin whether used in bathwater or as steam. For the former, pour a glass of ACV in a small basin containing warm water and use this as a refreshing face wash. If you want a deeper cleanse, put 3 tablespoons of ACV in a pan of just-boiled water, then lean your face over the pan while your head is covered with a towel for about 5 minutes. The steam will open up your pores and loosen any impurities within the surface of your skin. To finish up the cleanse, pat a cotton ball that has been soaked in ACV on the face to clean it.

Apple cider vinegar also relieves skin problems including hives, chicken pox, eczema, shingles, poison oak, diaper rash, psoriasis and poison ivy, just to mention a few. Simply soaking in an ACV bath will bring the needed relief.

Other uses

Learning about the many applications of apple cider vinegar has probably convinced you that it's a necessity for health maintenance, weight loss, and skincare. But those aren't the only benefits; you can also use ACV on your hair as a conditioner, to get rid of dandruff, to stop hair thinning and damage, to get rid of bald spots, to remove head lice, to cure itchy scalp, etc. You'll never run out of uses for apple cider vinegar in your everyday life!

Let's go over a few of these other uses of apple cider vinegar to give you just a glimpse of the healing power that this miracle cure holds.

As a remedy for dandruff and itching scalp

Flaking found in the skin of the scalp spells a common scalp condition called dandruff. Dandruff cases are neither serious nor contagious but it is imperative to treat them to avoid embarrassment and discomfort. Shampoo products catered to dandruff removal are available in the market, but they may not be as gentle or safe as you think they are. A mild case of dandruff may be treated by using a gentle hair cleanser or you can make your own version of a dandruff rinse using a cheap ingredient from the kitchen. Use apple cider vinegar! Do this by applying concentrated (undiluted) ACV to your hair or dry scalp, then massaging it well for several minutes; leave it on for up to an hour before rinsing.

As a remedy for bald spots

Bald spots as a skin disorder can affect both men and women. If you have this condition it is understandably difficult to remedy and can cause humiliation to some extent. There are many reasons for having such spots where hair is difficult to grow including hair loss, fungal infection, use of strong chemicals, to name a few. Finding a hard and permanent fix may be quite difficult but apple cider vinegar can be used to encourage healthy hair growth over the affected spot. With apple cider vinegar, get the other ingredients to make a nice solution to your hair growth dilemma. Squeeze out the juice from a pieced royal jelly capsule and mix it with 1 tablespoon of ACV. Apply it on the bald spots and leave it on overnight. Rinse in the morning.

To get rid of head lice

Are you experiencing a tickling feeling of something crawling in your hair? How about severe scalp itchiness? You will not be happy about this conclusion but there is a big possibility that you have head lice. And to have organisms like these resting on your crowning glory is enough to freak you out or ruin your day. To describe them, head lice are tiny, almost invisible, parasitic organisms that thrive among the hair strands in the head of humans. They are usually found in the scalp and some other parts of the body where hair is present. They feed of the blood of a host. You may want to get rid of them right away because they cause you to itch every time they draw blood from the scalp. There are over-the -counter medications available to kill head lice but you can also use apple cider vinegar just to avoid the chemical ingredients present in the preparations that are supplied by the pharmacy. Try using Apple Cider Vinegar or ACV. ACV has this active enzyme and antiseptic properties that kill bacteria causing itchy scalp as well as the parasites that may have been living in your luscious mane:

Ingredients

- Olive oil

- Lavender essential oil

- 1 cup of water

- 1 tablespoon of apple cider vinegar

Directions

Mix 3 parts of olive oil with 1 part of lavender essential oil. Saturate your scalp and hair with the mixture and cover with a shower cap for up to 5 hours. Mix ACV with water and use the mixture to rinse all the oil from your hair or scalp. You can then remove the nits and any remaining oil using a fine-tooth comb. Repeat the process over a period of up to 10 days or until you no longer see any more lice.

As a hair conditioner

The list of where to use apple cider vinegar continues. And this time, its application as a hair conditioner! Is it unbelievable? Well, you have no choice but to believe it. Apple cider vinegar is an excellent conditioner for the locks because it can leave your hair shiny without coating it with harmful chemicals like normal hair products can. Many commercial hair products do more harm than good for the hair because many of the ingredients are chemicals that may improve the appearance or texture of your hair, but leave damaging results if absorbed in the body. Some toxic chemicals are given harmless unsuspecting names. To name a few, artificial fragrances, methyl paraben, Propylene glycol, Methylisothiazolinone are just some of these harmful additives found in many shampoos and conditioner. To avoid exposing yourself to risks of cancer and other chemical-induced ailments, make the change to natural conditioners. All you need to get this done is to combine apple cider vinegar and filtered water; mix 4 parts of water with 1 part of ACV. Transfer the mixture to a spray bottle and mix the contents well. Divide your hair into small sections, then spray your conditioner on the scalp and hair starting from the roots and going up. Massage your hair and scalp and allow the mixture to sit for a few minutes before rinsing with water. If you don't like the smell of ACV, you may want to stay outdoors while you're waiting. Who could have known that the secret to clean and shiny hair is some vinegar in the kitchen. You'll know more once you give it a try.

CHAPTER 5:
SO HOW DO YOU MAKE YOUR OWN APPLE CIDER VINEGAR?

After reading through all the previous discussions, there is one thing that you should know. Apple cider vinegar has so many uses that there's probably at least one you're interested in trying yourself. Given that ACV is 100% organic and safe for consumption, you've got nothing to lose and everything to gain if it proves effective in resolving an issue that you've been struggling with for years. There are actually a lot of industrial apple cider vinegar products that you can choose from in the grocery aisle but many of which are not as healthy as you may think or resemble what real vinegar should be. There are some companies who do not produce pure and organic apple cider vinegar. In the United States for example, many companies can produce their own versions of apple cider vinegar without specific limits under the law since the law itself does not regulate what real apple cider vinegar must contain. Instead they use additives like colorants. The use of caramel colorants to mimic the color of real fermented ACV and sulfates for preservation. To make sure that you get the best of your apple cider vinegar choose the organic and natural ones. And for even more peace of mind about the process and what goes into the product, you can actually make ACV in the comfort of your own home! Especially if you live in places where there is a bounty source of apples, you will have an exact idea of what to do with your extra stock.

Apple cider vinegar is a product of fermentation—two types of fermentation, in fact. The process starts when you squeeze the liquid out of crushed apples. In the next stage, the sugars present in the juice are converted into alcohol by yeast. Then another round of fermentation takes place: the alcohol is converted into acetic acid by certain bacteria. You may not care how the process works, but if you're going to try it you'll want to be aware that it can take as long as three months. Through the three months of waiting, your very own homemade apple cider vinegar product will go through several processes with the end result of reducing raw and healthy apple cider vinegar. The recipes below will show you how to make ACV with both whole apples and apple scraps.

Making apple cider vinegar from whole apples

What you need:

- A piece of cheesecloth for covering the bowls

- 2 teaspoons of raw honey

- Chlorine-free water

- 10 apples (organically grown)

- 2 glass bowls (small and large)

Directions

First thing to do is to make sure that all ingredients are clean and ready. Wash the apples thoroughly, cut these into quarters, and let them air until they turn brown. Alternatively, you can core and peel the apples, eat the flesh, and use the next recipe to make ACV with the scraps. Place the browned apples into the smaller bowl, add the honey, mix well, and cover with water.

Prevent the apples from getting contaminated by foreign elements. Do this by finding something to seal the apples but allowing the natural flow of air inside the container. Cover the bowl with the cheesecloth and place it in a warm, dark place for up to 6 months (a hot water cupboard would be a good idea).

The next stage will be a bit confusing to those who are newbie to apple cider making but this stage is actually a crucial part of the process. By the time 6 months have passed, a grayish scum will have formed on the surface. Don't be scared, this is absolutely normal! This formation is what they call the "mother of vinegar", the very healthy aspect of apple cider vinegar. Rich in probiotics and enzymes, ACV's mother is also teeming with benefits. So do not discard these particles that accumulated while you allow the apple cider vinegar to ferment. You can spoon off the scum and the "mother" and add it to the other ingredients in your next batch. Once the liquid is strong enough for you, use a coffee filter to strain it, then transfer it to a clean container and leave it for an additional 4 to 6 weeks while covered with the cheesecloth. Finally, bottle it and store it in the refrigerator.

Making apple cider vinegar using scraps

The first process earlier discussed presented the technique of making apple cider vinegar using fresh and whole apples. This next recipe will present a way of reusing the peelings and parts of the apples that we normally throw away. Hence nothing is put to waste. This approach lets you make ACV from scraps— peels, bits and cores from organic apples. The end result is still apple cider vinegar in a raw and unpasteurized state, the perfect alternative to various health supplements.

What you need:

- A wide-mouth jar or a large bowl

- Apple scraps (browned)

- 2 tablespoons of raw honey

- A clean piece of cheesecloth to cover the bowl/jar to keep debris and flies off

- Chlorine-free water

Directions

Gather all the ingredients and materials that you will need. Place all the scraps in the jar/bowl, top it up with water, then add honey and stir well; ensure that the scraps are fully submerged. You can continue to add more scraps for several days if you want. To prevent the scraps from floating up, you can place a small jar inside the bigger jar. This way you can ensure that all apple scraps are submerged in the water to develop better flavor.

Make sure that no foreign organisms can enter the jar filled with your mixture. Cover the jar with the cheesecloth, place it in a warm, dark place and wait for it to ferment. Again, the cupboard containing your water heater would be a perfect place. You will start seeing the contents in the jar thickening after a few days and some grayish scum forming on top. The jar should also contain some sediments and the "mother". The mother need not be discarded because this is the healthy portion of the mixture.

At this point, you can spoon off the scum, stir the remaining liquid, and cover again; repeat the process for up to four weeks. Stop adding more scraps to the mixture; just leave it to ferment for a month, and then start tasting the resultant mixture. When it is strong enough for you, strain the liquid and transfer your ACV to a clean bottle or jar.

Remember, it is totally fine if your vinegar has a cloudy appearance. Real organic, unpasteurized, unfiltered and healthy apple cider vinegar need not be clear like those you see in the supermarket. The organic and healthy ACV will have impurities like sediments but these places the fermented vinegar at its healthiest state. Some sediment (the "mother") will probably remain. Just discard the scraps and place your homemade ACV in a refrigerator to stop the fermentation process. This is actually the best time to enjoy the goodness of apple cider vinegar. Use it in ways that pursue good health and long life.

Some important things to keep in mind when making ACV:

#1: Don't use metallic containers when making and or storing ACV. This will ensure that there will be no contamination while you ferment the apple cider vinegar. The acid present in the liquid will probably corrode any metallic items, resulting in contamination of the ACV. Stainless steel is the only metal that may be safe for use with ACV. It's better to use glass, wood or plastic containers (make sure that the glass doesn't have breaks or chips).

#2: When fermenting apple cider vinegar, be sure to keep the temperature within the range of 60-80 degrees F. Higher temperatures interfere with formation of "mother of vinegar", while lower temperatures will not produce a useful amount of ACV. For the mother to give the best benefits of the ACV it must not be exposed to high heat that can kill the good enzymes and probiotics in your homemade apple cider vinegar.

#3: Stir the mixture regularly to provide the oxygen needed for fermentation. Make sure that your hands are clean and the tools used in stirring are sterile. Using a cheesecloth filter allows the mixture to get enough oxygen since the cloth has spaces that let in air; don't use a lid. The oxygen will be used up by the good bacteria to transform the apples into apple cider vinegar in the process called aerobic respiration. For bacteria to produce acid it must also be allowed to breathe and in case of the organisms ACV they also need oxygen like we humans do.

How to use ACV

As you have learned throughout the book, you can use apple cider vinegar in many different ways, including diluting it in bath water, drinking it, adding it to food, and applying it on your skin. As a rule of thumb, dilute ACV before drinking it unless otherwise stated.

Tip: Don't be afraid of using the "mother"; it is actually the most nutritious part of apple cider vinegar. This quality makes ACV that includes the "mother" the most effective kind in terms of its therapeutic qualities. Impurities in apple cider vinegar will not affect the quality or the beneficial properties. It is even a sign that your apple cider vinegar is organic, raw and healthy for the body.

CONCLUSION

Key Takeaways

1. Apple cider vinegar can be used in virtually everything.

2. You can make your own apple cider vinegar for home use

3. You can stay healthy, lose weight, and make your hair and skin beautiful with ACV

4. Apple cider vinegar is effective if used properly and in moderation.

5. Always consult your doctor to inquire about any side effects if apple cider vinegar is taken with a prescribed medication or if you are pregnant or breastfeeding.

How To Put This Information Into Action

1. Identify a problem you are facing

2. Make your ACV using scraps or whole apples

3. Try using your homemade ACV to deal with the problem

4. Repeat the process!

5. The techniques provided are mere guides in the use of apple cider vinegar; do not ignore symptoms especially those that need special medical attention.

RESOURCES FOR FURTHER VIEWING AND READING

1. 15 Reasons to use apple cider vinegar:
   http://www.mindbodygreen.com/0-5875/15-Reasons-to-Use-Apple-Cider-Vinegar-Every-Day.html

2. Apple cider vinegar miracle for home and body:
   http://www.care2.com/greenliving/apple-cider-vinegar-miracle-for-home-and-body.html

3. Bragg Organic apple cider vinegar:
   http://bragg.com/products/bragg-organic-apple-cider-vinegar.html

4. 12 health benefits of apple cider vinegar:
   http://www.mnn.com/health/fitness-well-being/stories/12-health-benefits-of-apple-cider-vinegar

5. Health benefits of apple cider vinegar:
   http://www.eatingbirdfood.com/2012/02/health-benefits-of-apple-cider-vinegar-acv/

6. 10 Uses of apple cider you might not know:
   http://www.lifehack.org/articles/lifestyle/10-uses-of-apple-cider-vinegar-you-might-not-know-about.html

7. 15 Life hack Benefits of apple cider vinegar:
   http://www.lifehack.org/articles/lifestyle/15-benefits-apple-cider-vinegar.html

8. Interactions with other medications:
   http://naturaldatabase.therapeuticresearch.com/nd
   /PrintVersion.aspx?id=816&AspxAutoDetectCookie
   Support=1

Preview of "Modern Minimalism: How to Live with Less and Experience More in Today's Hectic World"

Consumerism Can Enslave Us

We live in a world where we are constantly looking for things we don't have simply because think we need them. Our lives have become empty as we fill the void with unnecessary stuff. We feel that getting the latest gadget and the trendiest clothes would ultimately make us happy because we feel accomplished by getting what we want. However, have you ever stopped to think about how soon the happiness fades away once we get what we wanted? Have you ever felt desiring another thing immediately after the purchase?

Humans have insatiable wants and needs. Abraham Maslow in his Hierarchy of Needs even concluded that a satisfied need is not a motivator of behavior, but directs us to move up to higher needs. Maslow emphasized that we can only have so much physiological needs – we need to move up to fulfilling needs such as relationships, self-esteem and self-actualization.

Have you ever thought of whether you actually need all the stuff you are constantly buying? For instance, you go and buy a large TV and subscribe to hundreds of premium TV channels thinking that you will no longer be missing your favorite TV shows. Then you buy the latest DVD player and sound system to match the new TV. Do you actually need to get all these to watch a show? In any case, how can you even watch all of the shows simultaneously? What follows is that you start with the hype of watching these shows then stop altogether because you run out of free time to sit back and relax. You become satiated, but you have to continue paying for these even when you don't even get the time to watch whatever you wanted to, because you slave away at work to pay for your mounting credit card, electric, and subscription bills. Tricky, isn't it?

This is the world of consumerism where we are meant to believe that we will live a happier life if we have certain things. Excessive buying may lead us to a point where none of the material things we obtain give us lasting inner happiness. We then become frustrated, depressed and feel as if we no longer know who we really are.

Do material things really make us happy? This is certainly debatable. What one person considers a need may not necessarily be a need for someone else. In fact, the situations are very different for different situations. Some of the stuff you need when you have a family may not be necessary when you are single. It is actually impossible to quantify happiness by comparing who is happier between two people. Actually, you don't have to live like a caveman to live a happy, healthy and fulfilling life. You just need balance.

Consumerism is an endless cycle that only makes us slaves of what we own. What we are exposed to in the society is what influences us to acquire the things we see. In fact, watching too much TV or surfing too much internet makes us less contented with what we already have, and more jealous of what others have. The glamour that comes with commercialization of literally everything sends us into a shopping mode where we think we must buy whatever we see on TV to feel contented with ourselves. However, this only fuels an insatiable desire to acquire more and more stuff that we end up not using; in fact, these stuff only stress us in trying to maintain them. Have you ever stopped to think if you are buying these items for your own benefit, or for the benefit of the manufacturer or seller?

Advertisements make us feel bad when we don't have some "essential things". Understanding the fundamental principles of minimalism can greatly affect the way we think, the way we interact with people and the level of satisfaction we derive from living a minimalist life.

To download the rest of this book, please click on the following link:

http://www.amazon.com/Modern-Minimalism-Experience-Minimalist-Lifestyle-ebook/dp/B00KU7DI20/ref=sr_1_1?ie=UTF8&qid=1403619202&sr=8-1&keywords=modern+minimalism

CHECK OUT MY OTHER BOOKS

If you're interested in finding my other books that are popular on Amazon and Kindle, simply click on the following link:

Below you'll find some of my other books that are popular on Amazon and Kindle as well. Simply click on the links below to check them out.

- **"Paleo Breakfast Recipes for Busy People: Quick & Easy Recipes to Help You Lose Weight, Feel Healthy and Look Amazing!"**

  Click the following link to check it out:

  http://www.amazon.com/Paleo-Breakfast-Recipes-Busy-People-ebook/dp/B00F3NC49O

- **"Food Addiction: A Proven Plan to Overcome Food Addiction for Life"**

  Click the following link to check it out:

  http://www.amazon.com/Food-Addiction-Overcome-Thinking-Obsessed-ebook/dp/B00EAUIUPS

- **"Thyroid Diet: A Natural Thyroid Solution Plan to Restoring Your Health in 30 Days or Less"**

  Click the following link to check it out:

  http://www.amazon.com/Thyroid-Diet-Solution-Restoring-Influenced-ebook/dp/B00EOAV6QY

- **"Irritable Bowel Syndrome: The Ultimate Guide to Eliminating IBS and Living a Healthier Life"**

Click the following link to check it out:

http://www.amazon.com/Irritable-Bowel-Syndrome-Eliminating-Healthier-ebook/dp/B00F4DHM3G

If the links do not work, for whatever reason, you can simply search for these titles on the Amazon website to find them.

ONE LAST THING

I want to sincerely thank-you for downloading my book.

I hope this book was able to help you to understand the hidden powder of apple cider vinegar in your everyday life. With this powerful homemade miracle cure, you will say goodbye to some of the challenges you have been going through including hair problems, skin problems, weight challenges, and other challenges related to your general health.

The next step is to make some apple cider vinegar and start using it to experience the benefits you have learned in the book!

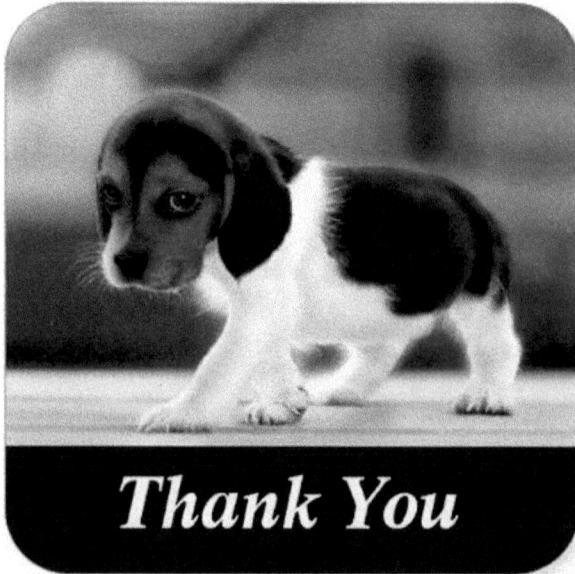

Thank You

If you enjoyed this book or feel that it has helped you in anyway, then could you please take a minute and post an honest review about it on Amazon?

Your review will help get my book out there to more people and they'll be forever grateful, as will I.

http://www.amazon.com/Apple-Cider-Vinegar-Beginners-Aromatherapy-ebook/product-reviews/B00LLO8ACO

OFFER FOR FREE BOOKS

If you're interested in receiving updates on new books and free book promotions, please click the link below:

https://docs.google.com/forms/d/1ttDqtdRjOeAEtA-BKnq5Hw668vjQSoVWcXCGQ8z9frA/viewform

www.ingramcontent.com/pod-product-compliance
Lightning Source LLC
Chambersburg PA
CBHW070029030426
42335CB00017B/2358